Study Guide & Activity Book

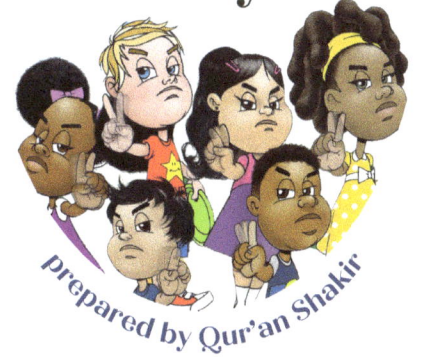

Study Guide for No Way, No How, I Say No!
Book by Dr. Qiana A. Johnson
Study Guide by Madame Q (Qur'an Shakir)

All rights reserved.

No part of this publication may be reproduced or transmitted in any form or by any means, electronic or mechanical, including photocopy, recording, or any information storage and retrieval system, without permission in writing from the copyright owner.

STUDY GUIDE No Way, No How, I Say No

ISBN: 979-8-9896332-9-6

Created, Edited and Designed by Qur'an Shakir

Published 2025 by BUBI - Building Us Beyond Imagination Publishing
sharingourlegacy@gmail.com

This workbook is a heartfelt thank you to Dr. Qiana A. Johnson for using her voice and expertise to protect and uplift young people.

It is a love offering to the brave souls who have found the courage to speak up, stand tall, and claim the protection they deserve —and to the caring adults who have taken action to keep children safe.

May this workbook empower every child to set boundaries with confidence and every adult to be a guardian of safety, ensuring that all children are surrounded by love, respect, and unwavering support.

PREFACE

Why This Study Guide?

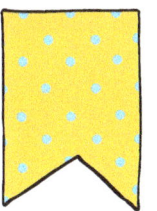

Child safety is one of the most pressing concerns facing families, educators, and caregivers today. According to the CDC, about 1 in 4 girls and 1 in 13 boys in the U.S. experience child sexual abuse at some point in childhood, and many cases go unreported due to fear, confusion, or a lack of awareness. In addition to sexual abuse, children face physical abuse, neglect, and emotional harm. These statistics reveal the urgent need to teach children about body safety and their right to say "No" in uncomfortable situations.

Being a mandated reporter, whether as a teacher, counselor, or childcare worker, requires us to be vigilant and proactive in protecting the children under our care. Mandated reporters are legally obligated to report any suspected abuse or neglect. However, reporting is only one part of the equation. To truly protect children, we must empower them to understand their rights and give them the tools to speak up when something doesn't feel right.

No Way, No How, I Say No! by Dr. Qiana A. Johnson addresses the critical need for body safety education by putting children at the center of the conversation. This book helps young readers understand their autonomy, offering them the language to express discomfort and assert boundaries. Written in a playful and rhythmic way, it engages children in a way that feels approachable yet impactful, making it easier to discuss sensitive topics like body boundaries and inappropriate touch.

This study guide is designed to take the message of the book further, providing parents, educators, and caregivers with a structured approach to teaching body safety. It offers activities, discussions, and assessments that reinforce the book's lessons, helping children internalize what it means to set boundaries, say "No," and reach out to trusted adults.

The need for a study guide like this goes beyond simply educating children on the mechanics of safety. It also fosters an environment where children feel empowered and confident to use their voice. By creating spaces for open dialogue, providing role-playing exercises, and using a combination of creative and reflective activities, this curriculum supports children in developing a strong sense of self-advocacy.

In a world where too many children experience abuse, this book and study guide serve as powerful tools for prevention. As we work together—parents, educators, and communities—we can build a culture where children understand that their bodies belong to them and that they have the right to say "No, no way, no how."

It is my hope that in addition to supporting children in their journey toward body safety, this study guide will also equip adults with the knowledge, language, and courage to foster open communication and create safer environments for all children.

With all sincerity,

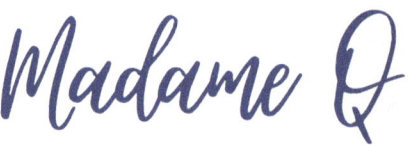

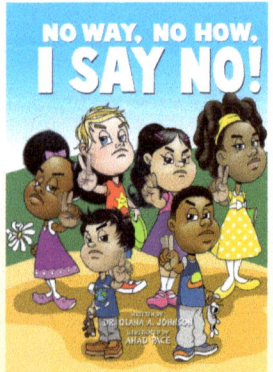

This study guide is prepared with the permission of author, Dr. Qiana A. Johnson, as an accompaniment to her book No Way, No How, I Say No!

Message to those using this study guide and curriculum plans

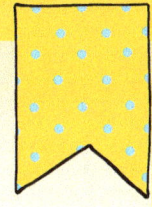

Dear Educators, Parents, Caregivers, and Community Leaders,

Thank you for choosing to engage with No Way, No How, I Say No! by Dr. Qiana A. Johnson and this accompanying study guide and curriculum plan. You are taking a vital step in empowering children to understand their bodies, establish boundaries, and foster a sense of safety and confidence in their interactions with others.

This guide is designed to provide you with practical tools and engaging activities to facilitate meaningful conversations about body safety and consent. By integrating these lessons into your discussions, you are helping children recognize their rights and encouraging them to trust their instincts when faced with uncomfortable situations.

As you navigate through the activities and questions, remember that your role as a trusted adult is essential in shaping a child's understanding of their own body and the importance of respectful interactions. Your guidance can make a lasting impact, helping them to develop the courage to speak up and the awareness to protect themselves.

Together, we can create a supportive environment where children feel safe, valued, and empowered. Thank you for your commitment to nurturing the next generation's understanding of body safety and consent.

With gratitude and prayer,

BUBI - Building Us Beyond Imagination Enterprises Publishing

WHAT THE DATA SHOWS

In 2016, 57,329 children were victims of sexual abuse in the United States.

Every 68 seconds, an American is sexually assaulted. And every 9 minutes, that victim is a child. Meanwhile, only 25 out of every 1,000 perpetrators will end up in prison.

One in 9 girls and 1 in 20 boys under the age of 18 experience sexual abuse or assault.

- 82% of all victims under 18 are female.
- Females ages 16-19 are 4 times more likely than the general population to be victims of rape, attempted rape, or sexual assault.

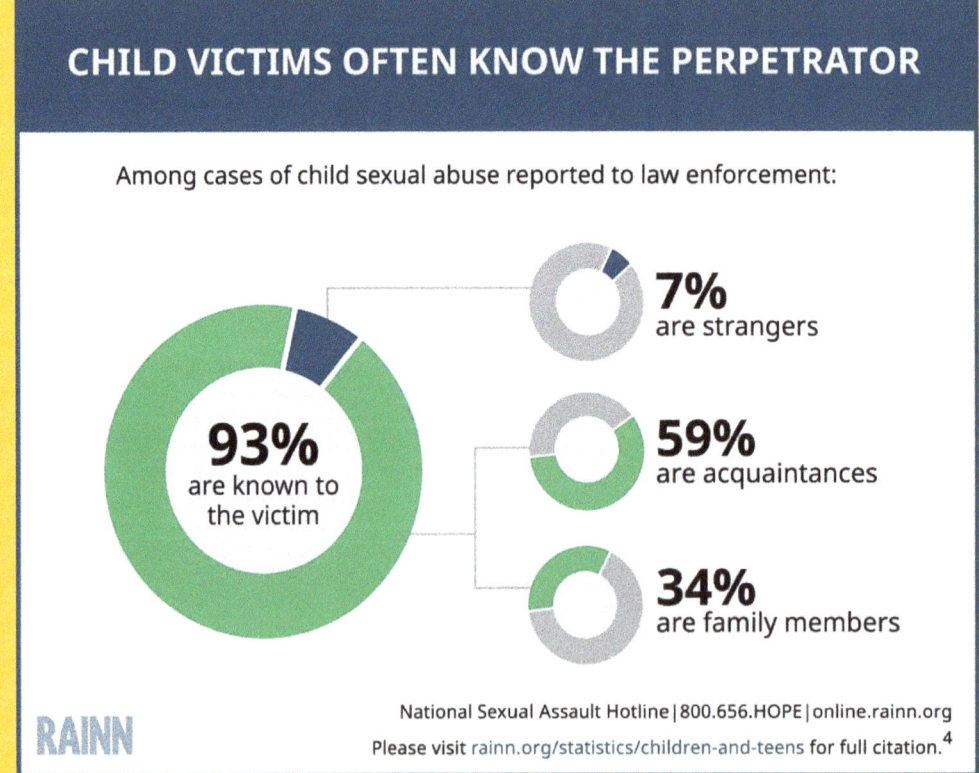

CHILD VICTIMS OFTEN KNOW THE PERPETRATOR

Among cases of child sexual abuse reported to law enforcement:

- 93% are known to the victim
- 7% are strangers
- 59% are acquaintances
- 34% are family members

National Sexual Assault Hotline | 800.656.HOPE | online.rainn.org
Please visit rainn.org/statistics/children-and-teens for full citation.[4]

RAINN

Information gathered from www.rainn.org

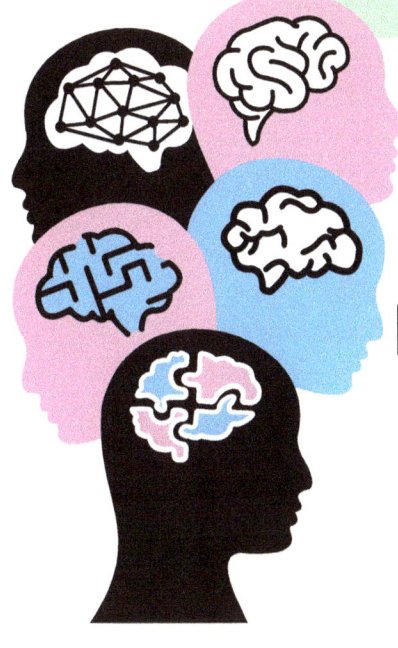

The effects of child sexual abuse can be long-lasting and affect the victim's mental health.

Victims are more likely than non-victims to experience the following mental health challenges:

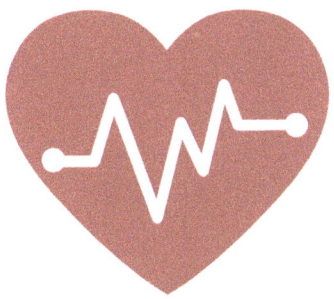

- About 4 times more likely to develop symptoms of drug abuse
- About 4 times more likely to experience PTSD as adults
- About 3 times more likely to experience a major depressive episode as adults

OVERVIEW: - TYPES OF SEXUAL ABUSE

Sexual Harassment

You should be able to feel comfortable in your place of work or learning. If you are being sexually harassed, you can report it to the authorities at your job, school, or local law enforcement.

Stalking

Learn more about stalking behaviors to help you notice them before they escalate—and take steps to protect yourself.

Sexual Assault

intentionally touching another person in a sexual manner, without that person's consent

Child Sexual Abuse

sexual activity that happens to a person under the age of 18 and is unwanted or involves pressure, manipulation, bullying, intimidation, threats, deception or force

Adult Survivors of Child Sexual Abuse

perpetrator of sexual abuse in a position of trust or responsible for the child's care, such as a family member, teacher, clergy member, coach, or other children such as older siblings

Using Technology to Hurt Others

Some people use technology, such as digital photos, videos, apps, and social media, to engage in harassing, unsolicited, or non-consensual sexual interactions

Information gathered from www.rainn.org

OVERVIEW: - TYPES OF SEXUAL ABUSE

Sexual Abuse by Medical Professionals

When you go to the doctor, dentist, hospital or physical therapist, or see other medical professionals, you trust them to treat you with respect as they care for your health

Sexual Exploitation by Helping Professionals

Sexual exploitation by a helping professional is a serious violation of trust and, in many cases, the law

Multiple-Perpetrator Sexual Assault

Multiple-perpetrator sexual assault, sometimes called gang rape, occurs when two or more perpetrators act together to sexually assault the same victim

Elder Abuse

As the number of older adults in America increases, it will become all the more important to be aware of the warning signs of elder abuse

Sexual Abuse of People with Disabilities

Consent is crucial when any person engages in sexual activity, but it plays an even bigger, and more complicated role when someone has a disability.

Legal Role of Consent

The legal definitions for terms like rape, sexual assault, and sexual abuse vary from state to state. Consent often plays an important role in determining whether an act is legally considered a crime.

Information gathered from www.rainn.org

OVERVIEW: - TYPES OF SEXUAL ABUSE

Prisoner Rape

An inmate, a former inmate, or know an inmate who survived sexual assault while in prison, there are resources available.

Military Sexual Trauma

Military Sexual Trauma, or MST, is the term used by the Department of Veteran Affairs to describe the effects of sexual violence experienced by a military Service member.

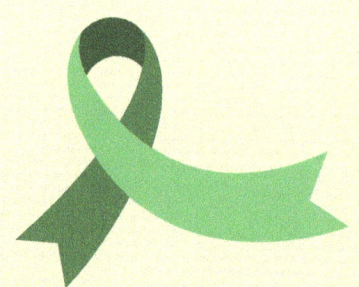

Information gathered from www.rainn.org

Recognizing Possible Warning Signs of Abuse

It's important for parents, caregivers, teachers, and community members to recognize possible warning signs of abuse in children. While these signs do not always indicate abuse, they can be red flags that a child may need help.

PHYSICAL SIGNS
- Unexplained injuries – bruises, burns, cuts, or fractures with no clear explanation.
- Frequent complaints of pain – headaches, stomach aches, or pain in private areas.
- Wearing inappropriate clothing – long sleeves or pants in hot weather (to cover injuries).
- Discomfort sitting or walking – possible sign of physical or sexual abuse.

BEHAVIORAL CHANGES
- Sudden fearfulness or anxiety – fear of a particular person or place.
- Loss of interest in activities – withdrawing from friends, school, or hobbies.
- Regression – bedwetting, thumb-sucking, or other younger behaviors returning.
- Excessive secrecy – refusing to talk about certain topics or avoiding discussions about safety.
- Increased aggression or mood swings – acting out, being overly defensive, or showing extreme anger.

SOCIAL AND EMOTIONAL SIGNS
- Difficulty trusting others – hesitation to be around adults or sudden clinginess.
- Low self-esteem or self-blame – making negative comments about themselves.
- Avoidance of physical contact – flinching, pulling away, or refusing to be touched.
- Fear of being left alone – expressing distress when separated from a caregiver.

WARNING SIGNS IN COMMUNICATION & PLAY
- Talking about "secrets" or "bad things" happening – vague statements that may indicate abuse.
- Using language or knowledge about sexual topics beyond their age – may indicate exposure to inappropriate behavior.
- Reenacting disturbing scenarios in play – using dolls or toys to act out concerning events.

SIGNS IN SCHOOL PERFORMANCE & DAILY LIFE
- Sudden drop in grades – difficulty concentrating, losing motivation.
- Frequent absences – avoiding school or daycare.
- Eating/sleeping disturbances – loss of appetite, nightmares, or difficulty sleeping.

WHAT TO DO IF YOU NOTICE THESE SIGNS
- ✅ Listen carefully – If a child talks about something troubling, stay calm and listen.
- ✅ Reassure them – Let them know they are not to blame and that you are there to help.
- ✅ Do not pressure them to talk – Instead, gently ask open-ended questions like, "Can you tell me more about that?"
- ✅ Report your concerns – If you suspect abuse, contact the appropriate authorities (child protective services, a school counselor, or a trusted professional).

Recognizing these signs early can help protect children and ensure they receive the support they need. If you suspect abuse, take action—your response could make all the difference.

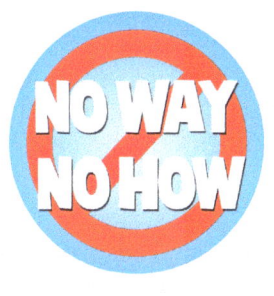

How to Talk to Children to Keep Them Safe

Talking about body safety doesn't have to be scary—it should be empowering! Keep the conversation open, honest, and age-appropriate to build trust and awareness.

1. Use the Proper Names for Body Parts
- Teach children the correct terms for their private parts (e.g., penis, vagina, vulva, buttocks, breasts) just like any other body part.
- This helps reduce shame and confusion and makes it easier for them to report abuse if necessary.
    - Example:
        - "Just like your arms and legs have names, your private parts have names too. They are called _____."

2. Teach Body Autonomy & Boundaries
- Help children understand that their body belongs to them, and they have the right to say "No" to unwanted touch.
- Reinforce that safe adults respect their "No."
    - Example:
        - "If you don't want a hug or a high five, that's okay! You get to decide who touches you."

3. Explain the Difference Between Safe & Unsafe Touch
- Teach that some touches are okay (like a hug from a loved one when they want it) and some are not okay (like touching private parts).
- Emphasize that no one should touch their private parts unless it's for health or hygiene (e.g., a doctor with a parent present).
    - Example:
        - "A safe touch makes you feel good and comfortable, like a hug from grandma. An unsafe touch makes you feel confused or uncomfortable."

5. Encourage Open Communication
- Let children know they can talk to you about anything without fear of getting in trouble.
- Assure them that they will always be believed and protected.
    - Example:
        - "If anyone makes you feel uncomfortable, even if they say it's a secret, you can always tell me. You will never be in trouble."

How NOT to Talk to Children About Private Parts and Safety

1. Don't Blame or Question Their Timing
- Avoid saying: "Why didn't you tell me sooner?" or "Why did you wait so long to say something?"
- These questions can make a child feel guilty, ashamed, or afraid to speak up in the future.
    - Instead, reassure the child that they are not at fault and that they are safe and supported. Say:
        - "I'm so glad you told me. You did the right thing, and I'm here to help."
        - "Thank you for trusting me. You are very brave for sharing this with me."

2. Don't Use Nicknames for Private Parts
- Using pet names can confuse children and make it harder for them to report abuse clearly.

3. Don't Instill Fear Instead of Confidence
- Fear-based teaching can cause anxiety instead of empowerment.
    - Example: "Strangers are dangerous!" should be replaced with "Most people are kind, but some may try to trick you, so always tell me if something feels wrong."

4. Don't Force Physical Affection
- Allow children to decide how they want to show affection.
    - Example: "Go hug your uncle! It's rude if you don't." Instead, say "Would you like to wave or high-five instead?"

5. Don't Ignore Their Feelings
- Always listen when a child expresses discomfort or shares an experience.

6. Don't Keep Conversations One-Time Only
- Make it an ongoing conversation! Find natural ways to bring up body safety in daily life.

Overview:

No Way, No How, I Say No! empowers children to take control of their bodies and confidently say "no" to any form of inappropriate touching or behavior. Through engaging rhymes and simple language, the book helps children recognize their boundaries, trust their instincts, and feel safe speaking up. This guide provides activities, discussion questions, and key learning points to reinforce the book's important lessons.

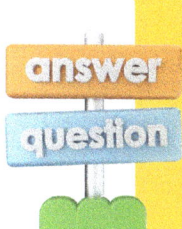

OBJECTIVES

- Understand Body Safety: Teach children that their bodies belong to them, and they have the right to say "no" to anything that makes them uncomfortable.
- Recognize Boundaries: Help children learn to set clear boundaries and identify trusted adults and safe spaces they can turn to for sharing concerns.
- Empowerment: Build children's confidence in speaking up for themselves without fear.
- **Body Autonomy:**
  - Children learn that their bodies belong to them, and they have the right to control who touches them.
- **Empowerment Through the Five Senses:**
  - The story explores how children can use their senses—sight, hearing, taste, smell, and touch—to protect themselves and express boundaries.
- **Saying No with Confidence:**
  - The rhyme empowers children to stand up for themselves and say "No" to unwanted touch, requests, or situations that feel wrong.
- **Seeking Help:**
  - Reinforces the importance of telling a trusted adult if they feel uncomfortable or unsafe.

KEY THEMES

- Body Ownership
- Boundaries and Consent
- Trusting Feelings and Instincts
- Empowerment to Speak Up
- Body Safety Using the Five Senses

Pre-Reading Activity:

Key Vocabulary

Below are some of the key vocabulary words children should learn and know.

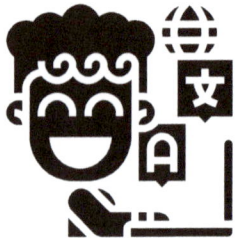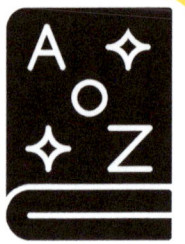

These words help empower children to understand their right to body safety and how to communicate effectively when setting boundaries.

Vocabulary	Definition
Boundaries	Limits that you set to protect yourself
Consent / Permission	Saying "yes" to allow someone to do something; it's okay to say "no" if you don't want to
Empowerment	Feeling strong and confident about making choices for yourself
Privacy	Keeping certain things to yourself, like when you go to the bathroom or change clothes; no one should invade your privacy.
Private Parts	Parts of your body that are covered by your bathing suit
Respect	Treating others kindly and understanding that everyone's body and feelings are important.
Secret	Something that is hidden or not told to others; some secrets are not okay to keep, especially if they make you feel bad or unsafe
Trusted Adult	Someone you feel safe with, like a parent, teacher, or family member.
Touch	Any contact with your body, such as a hug or handshake; there are safe touches and unsafe touches.

Pre-Reading Activities
Choice Board

Children May Enjoy These Activities Before Reading the Book:

These pre-reading activities will help children feel more engaged and prepared to dive into the lessons of No Way, No How, I Say No! while reinforcing important concepts of body safety and boundaries.

Introduce Body Boundaries with a Visual Activity

- Materials: Large paper, markers, stickers
- Activity: Draw an outline of a person on a large piece of paper and ask the children to help identify "public" and "private" areas of the body. You can use stickers or colored markers to highlight safe touch zones and areas that should remain private. This introduces the idea of body boundaries in a visual and interactive way.

What is Consent?

- Discussion: Start by explaining the concept of consent. Use examples like, "If you want to borrow a toy, do you ask permission first?" This helps children understand that consent is about asking permission and respecting other people's answers.
- Interactive: Have the children practice giving or denying consent through simple role-playing. For example, one child asks, "Can I borrow your crayon?" and the other practices saying "Yes" or "No" with confidence.

Five Senses Exploration

- Activity: Help children name their five senses (sight, hearing, touch, taste, and smell). Discuss how each sense helps them interact with the world and keep them safe. Ask questions like, "What do your eyes help you see?" or "How do your ears help you hear?"
- Game: Play a game where children identify objects using their senses. For example, use a blindfold to have them feel or smell an object and guess what it is. This connects to the book's focus on the five senses for safety.

Story Prediction

- Discussion: Show the cover of the book and ask the children to predict what the story might be about. Ask questions like, "What do you think the characters will say 'No' to?" or "Why do you think it's important to say 'No' sometimes?"
- Engage Curiosity: Encourage them to think about times they've said "No" and why it was important. This can lead to a discussion on when it's okay to say "No" to protect themselves.

Safe and Unsafe Touch Sorting Game

- Materials: Cards with various actions. Create on index cards, one action on each card. Sample actions can be "a hug from a parent, a pat on the back from a teacher, someone touching your private parts, a handshake, a high five".
- Activity: Children sort the cards into two categories: "Safe" and "Unsafe" touch. This activity introduces them to appropriate versus inappropriate touch in a simple, hands-on way.

Emotion Charades

- Activity: Play a game of charades where children act out different emotions (happy, sad, scared, angry).
- Discuss how these emotions relate to how they feel when someone touches them in a way they don't like. Help them understand that if they feel uncomfortable or scared, it's okay to say "No" and seek help.

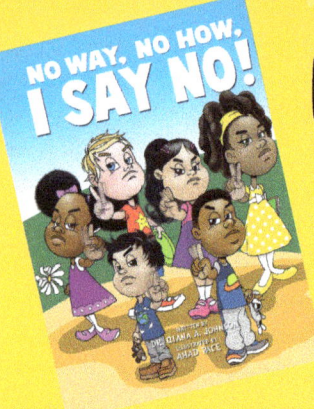

BODY SAFETY QUESTIONS
No Way, No How, I Say No!

Use these questions to help children start thinking about body safety in a way that feels natural and encourages them to open up.

01.
What are your "safe zones" on your body, and who is allowed to touch them?

02.
What would you do if someone touched you in a way that made you uncomfortable?

03.
Who are trusted adults you can go to if you ever feel unsafe or uncomfortable?

04.
Explore your feelings and instincts. How do you know when something is wrong or unsafe?

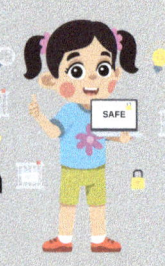

05.
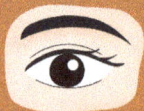
What should you do if someone asks you to keep a secret about touching?

06.
Explain why it is important to speak up if something makes you feel uncomfortable.

07.
How can you help a friend if they feel unsafe or scared about their body?

These questions foster open dialogue, build confidence in expressing feelings, and teach children the importance of body safety and boundaries

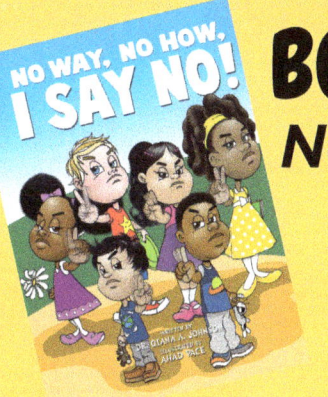

BODY SAFETY QUESTIONS
No Way, No How, I Say No!

Use these questions to help children start thinking about body safety in a way that feels natural and encourages them to open up.

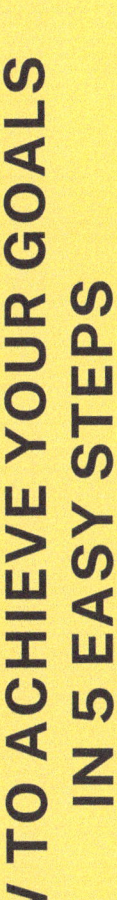

HOW TO ACHIEVE YOUR GOALS IN 5 EASY STEPS

01 What are your "safe zones" on your body, and who is allowed to touch them?

02 What would you do if someone touched you in a way that made you uncomfortable?

03 Who are trusted adults you can go to if you ever feel unsafe or uncomfortable?

04 Explore your feelings and instincts. How do you know when something is wrong or unsafe?

05 What should you do if someone asks you to keep a secret about touching?

06 Explain why it is important to speak up if something makes you feel uncomfortable.

@reallygreatsite

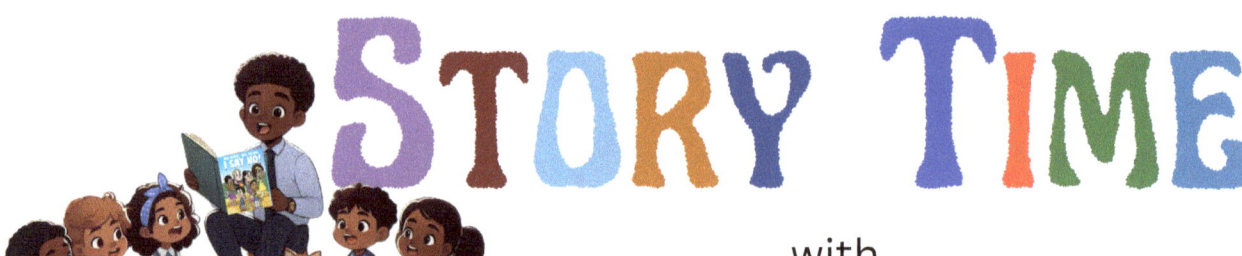

Story Time

with

No Way, No How, I Say No!

Engage children in an interactive and meaningful story time that reinforces the lessons of body safety, consent, and personal boundaries in a fun and age-appropriate way.

1. Gather children to sit in a circle.
2. Before reading, examine the cover. Ask questions:
    a. Have you ever been in a situation where you had to say "No"? How did it feel?
    b. Why is it important to be able to say "No" when something doesn't feel right?
    c. Who are the trusted adults in your life that you can talk to if something makes you uncomfortable?
    d. If you wrote a book about saying "No," what would you put on the cover?
3. Read the book aloud with enthusiasm and different voices for the characters.
4. Pause to ask engaging questions:
    a. "How does this character feel?"
    b. "What would you do in this situation?"
5. Let the children chant the reframe with you.....
6. Reinforce boundary-setting in a safe, engaging way after reading.
    a. Call up volunteers to act out different scenarios while the group practices saying, "No way, no how, I say no!"
        i. Sample scenarios:
            1. Someone tries to give a hug when the child doesn't want one.
            2. A trusted adult asks before giving a high-five.
            3. A friend asks to see private parts.
7. At the end, they all celebrate knowing safe ways to be an advocate for themselves

Empowerment Affirmation
(2-3 minutes)

Stand together in a circle and repeat:
- "My body is mine, and I have the power to say no!"
- "I am brave, I am strong, and I will always tell a trusted adult!"

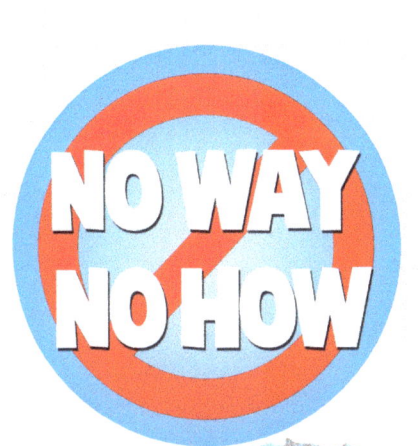

Use this affirmation after reading the book No Way, No How, I Say No! by Dr. Qiana Johnson or to begin activities and sessions with children.

After reading   **Activities:**

Body Safety Chart

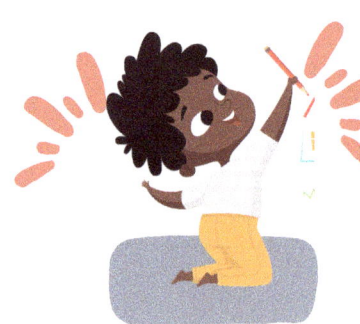

Create a chart with the five senses and ask the children to list ways they can use each sense to stay safe. For example, "My ears can hear if someone says something wrong."

Role-Playing Scenarios:

Act out simple scenarios where a child might need to say "no." For example, "Someone tries to show you a picture of a private part." Encourage children to practice saying "No way, no how, I say no!"

Draw Your Safe Zone:

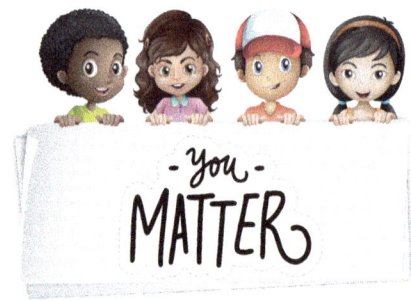

Have children draw an outline of their bodies and color in the parts they consider "private" or off-limits. This visual activity reinforces the concept of body boundaries.

Create a "No" Sign:

Have the children create their own "No Way, No How, I Say No!" signs using markers and paper. Let them decorate it to make it personal and empowering.

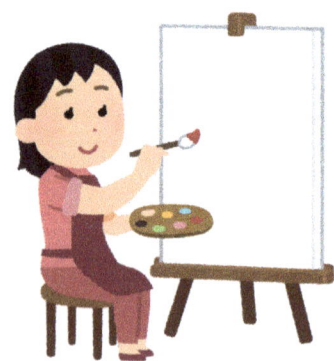

Sample

Role Playing Scenarios

for Teaching Children to Say "No"

These scenarios provide children with opportunities to practice using clear, firm words to assert their boundaries and prioritize their safety.

Scenario: An Unwanted Hug

Situation: A family friend tries to give the child a hug, but the child feels uncomfortable.

Role-Playing Response: Teach the child to say, "No, thank you, I don't want a hug right now," and step back or use a hand gesture to signal their boundary.

Scenario: Being Asked to Keep a Secret

Situation: An older child or adult tells the child, "This is our little secret," after doing or saying something that makes the child uncomfortable.

Role-Playing Response: Encourage the child to say, "I don't keep secrets like this. I'm going to tell a trusted adult."

Scenario: Peer Pressure to Look at Inappropriate Pictures

Situation: A friend or classmate asks the child to look at inappropriate images on a phone or device.

Role-Playing Response: Help the child practice saying, "No, I don't want to look at that. It's not okay," and walking away to tell a trusted adult.

Scenario: An Adult Asking for Help with Private Tasks

Situation: An adult asks the child to help them with something private, like changing clothes or cleaning up inappropriately.

Role-Playing Response: Teach the child to say, "No, I'm not allowed to do that. I'll get someone else to help you."

Scenario: Being Offered Something Unsafe to Taste or Smell

Situation: Someone offers the child a strange drink, food, or substance and pressures them to try it.

Role-Playing Response: Practice with the child saying, "No, I don't want to try that. I need to tell my parent or teacher," and refusing to take it.

After reading Activities

My Body, My Rules Poster:

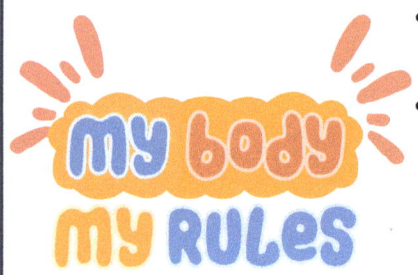

- Materials: Poster board, markers, stickers.
- Instructions: Have the children create a "My Body, My Rules" poster.
  - They can draw themselves and write down rules that they decide about their own bodies, like "I decide who hugs me" or "I can say no if I feel uncomfortable."

Role Play:

- Instructions: Partner children up for a role-playing activity where one person says "No" to an unwanted action (e.g., a hug or touch). This builds confidence in practicing saying "No" in a safe environment.
- Discussion: After the role play, discuss how it felt to say "No" and how important it is to mean what you say.

Sense Match-Up Game:

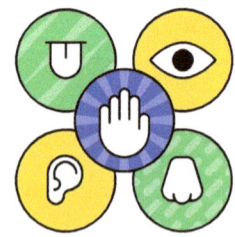

- Instructions: Create cards with different scenarios involving sight, sound, touch, smell, and taste. Ask the children to match the scenario with the correct sense and discuss how they can use that sense to keep themselves safe.
- Example: "Someone shows you a picture of a private part" (Sight) → What should you do? Say, "No, I don't want to see that."

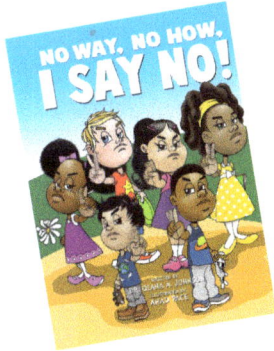

DISCUSSION QUESTIONS

PRIVATE PARTS:

- What does it mean when the book says, "This is my body and I say no"?
  - Encourage children to talk about how they control who can or cannot touch their bodies.

BODY OWNERSHIP:

- Who can you go to if someone makes you feel unsafe?
- Guide them to identify safe adults in their lives, such as parents, teachers, or guardians.
- Can you name some safe people you would tell if someone touched you inappropriately or said something inappropriate to you?

FIVE SENSES AND SAFETY:

- How do the five senses help the characters in the book stay safe? For example, how do their eyes, ears, or hands help them decide what feels right?
- Why is it important to use your eyes, ears, mouth, nose, and hands to stay safe?

SPEAKING UP

- How does it feel to say "no" when something isn't right? Why is it important to speak up?
- What does it mean to say "No way, no how, I say no"?
- Discuss how this phrase empowers children to set boundaries and protect themselves.
- What would you do if someone tried to touch you in a way that makes you uncomfortable?
- Encourage children to practice what they would do in these situations.
- Talk about how being brave can help them protect themselves and others.

PRIVATE PARTS:

- Have discussion with children about the anatomically correct names of their private body parts.
- Why is it important to protect your private parts, and what should you do if someone wants to touch or see them?
- Reinforce that private parts are not for others to see or touch, and it's always okay to say "no."

Creative Activity

My Safety Superpower Craft

This activity will help children internalize
body safety lessons through creativity.
(10 minutes)

Materials: Paper, crayons, stickers
How to Play:
- Have children draw themselves as a superhero of safety with their special power of saying NO!
- Encourage them to write or dictate one safety rule they learned.

Reflection JOURNAL

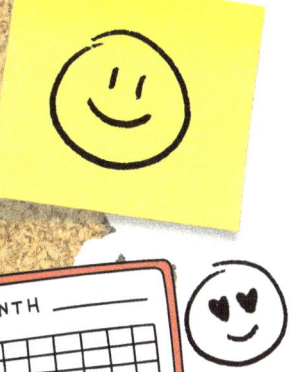
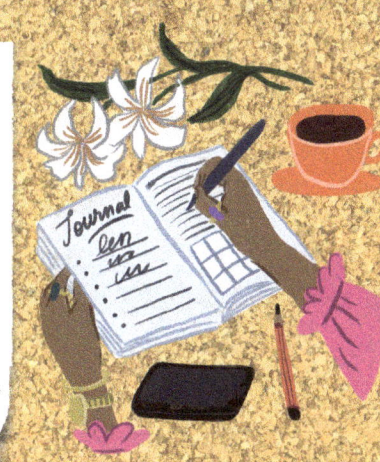

Write or draw a situation where you felt uncomfortable, and how you responded. If you haven't experienced this, imagine how you would say "No way, no how, I say no."

Think about a time when you said "No" to something small, like refusing a hug or choosing not to do something you didn't feel like doing. How did it feel to say "No"? Write about why it's important to practice saying "No" when something doesn't feel right.

This week, practice saying "No" when you don't feel like doing something, like giving a hug or playing a game. How did it feel to set your boundaries?

Write about why it's important to tell an adult when something makes you feel unsafe or uncomfortable. How do you feel after sharing your worries with someone you trust?

Write about who your trusted adults are and how they make you feel safe. How would you start the conversation if you needed to tell them about something that didn't feel right?

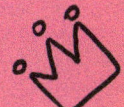

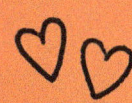

Write about a time when you said "No" and how the other person reacted. How did it make you feel to stand up for yourself? What can you do to feel even more confident in saying "No" when something doesn't feel right?

What are some ways you can practice setting boundaries in your daily life to help you feel more confident?

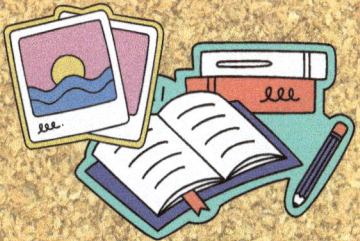

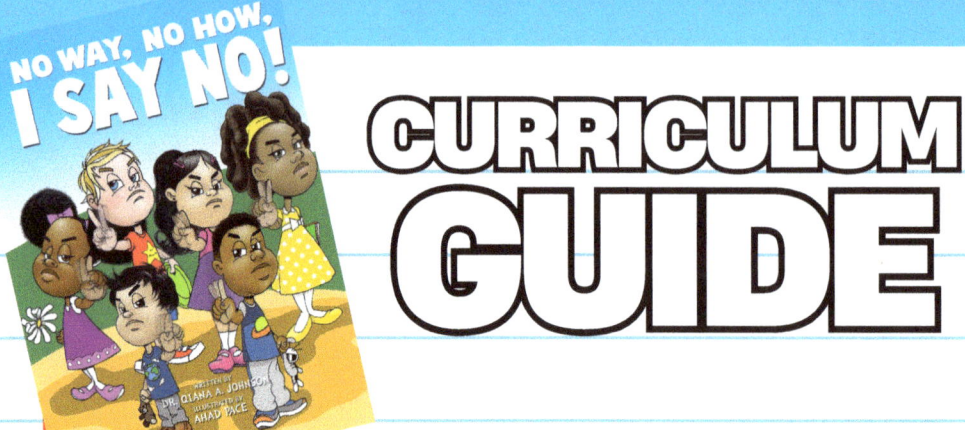

CURRICULUM GUIDE

Curriculum Overview:

Here is a six-week curriculum plan for studying No Way, No How, I Say No! by Dr. Qiana A. Johnson. This curriculum is designed to teach children about body safety, boundaries, and respect for themselves and others.

Using the book's rhyming verses and the five senses as a guide, students will explore important lessons about consent, private parts, and the power of saying "No."

Lessons are interactive and age-appropriate, fostering communication and trust between children and their trusted adults.

A body safety quiz follows the curriculum plan.

Our prayer is that this curriculum ensures that children understand the lessons in No Way, No How, I Say No! and feel empowered to use them in their everyday lives.

Week 1:
Introduction to Body Safety

Objective:
- Understand that everyone has control over their own body and the right to say "No."
- Help children understand that their bodies are their own, and they have the right to decide who can touch, see, or interact with their body.

Activity:
- Read the introduction of No Way, No How, I Say No! as a class.
- Discuss the concept of personal boundaries and what it means to say "No" to unwanted touch.

Discussion Questions:
- What does it mean to say "No" when someone wants to touch you?
- Why is it important to have control over your own body?

Activity:
Create a "My Body, My Rules" poster where children write or draw examples of when they can say "No" to something that makes them uncomfortable.

Use body outlines for children to color, marking their "private zones" that no one else should touch.

Homework: Write down three safe adults you can talk to if you feel unsafe.

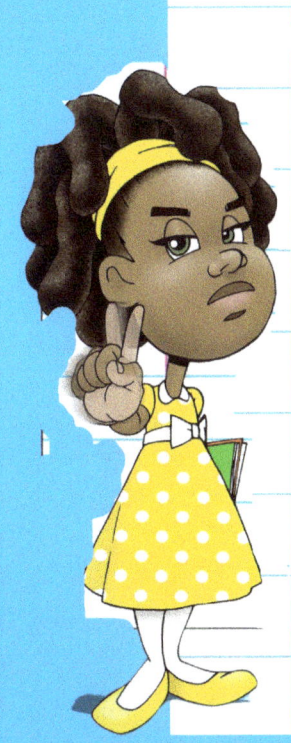

Color and mark your "private zones" that no one else should touch.

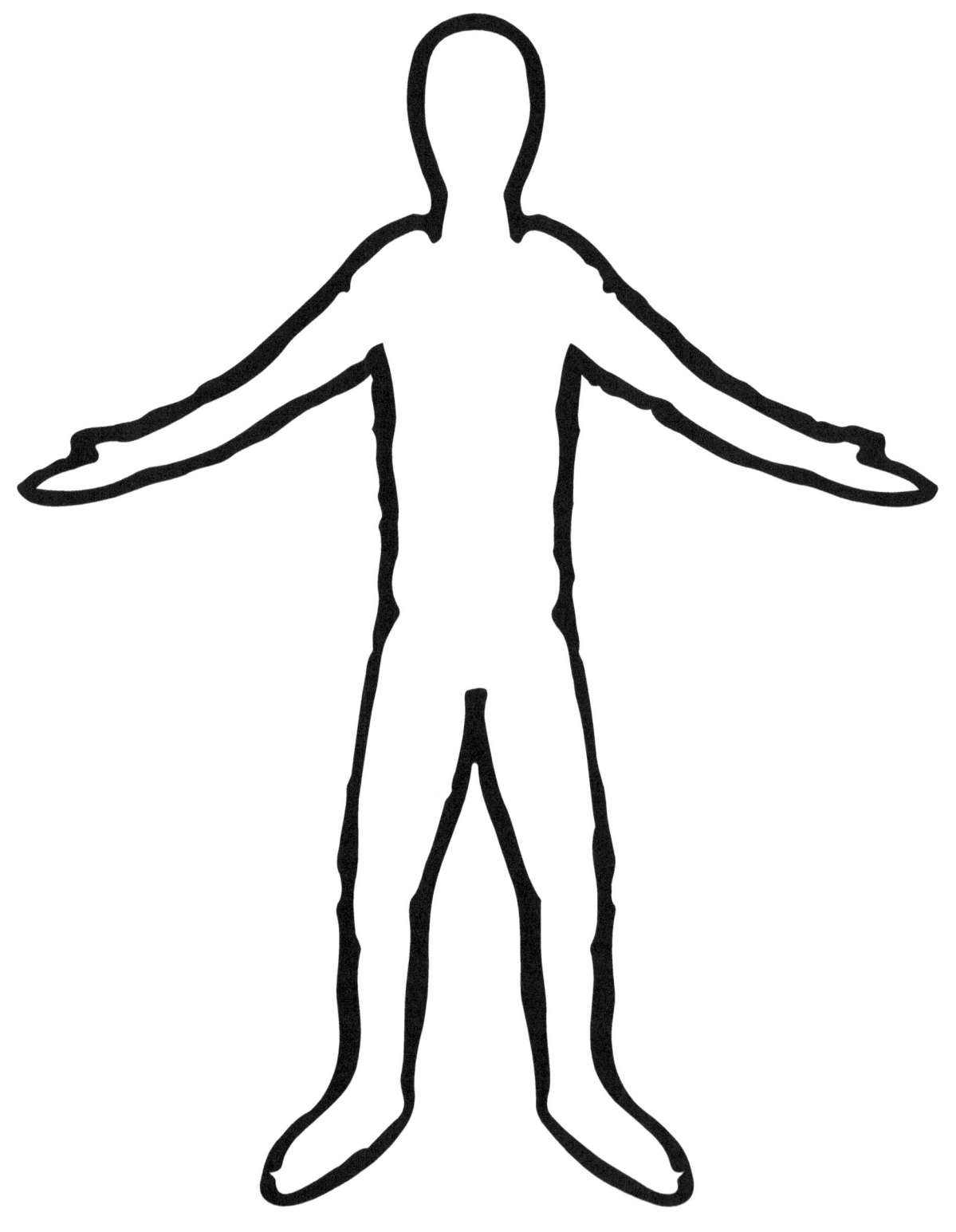

Write down three safe adults you can talk to if you feel unsafe.

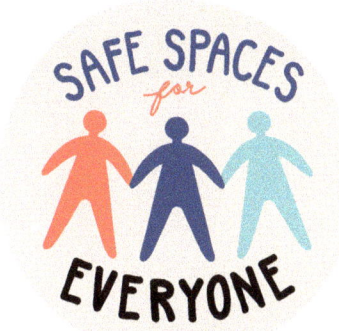

Write down three safe adults you can talk to if you feel unsafe.

✅ _____

✅ _____

✅ _____

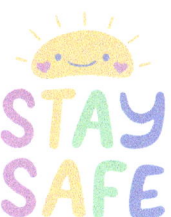

Week 2:
The Five Senses & Boundaries

Objective:
- Learn how each sense helps identify safe and unsafe situations.
- Help children understand their five senses and how they can use them to protect themselves.

Activity: Reread key sections of the book where the five senses (eyes, ears, mouth, nose, fingers) are discussed.

Discussion Questions:
- How do your eyes help you set boundaries about what you want to see?
- Why is it important to listen to words that make you feel safe?
- What kinds of things should we say "No" to seeing, hearing, or touching?
- How can we use our senses to know when something feels wrong?

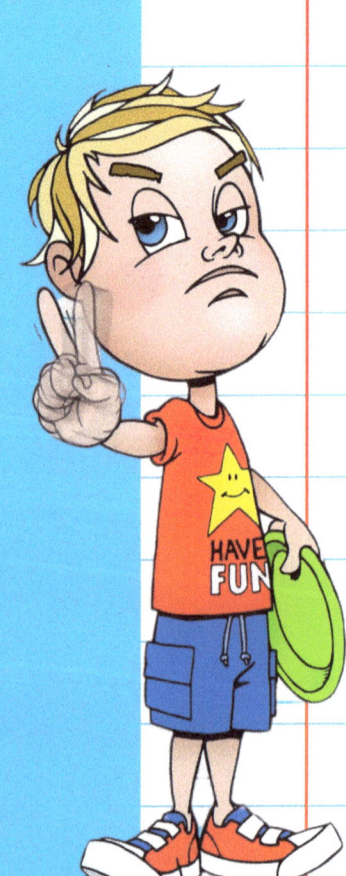

Activity:
- Have students draw a picture of their five senses and label how each one helps them know when something is wrong or makes them uncomfortable.
- Sensory matching game: Match pictures of the senses (eye, ear, mouth, etc.) with safe and unsafe scenarios.
- Draw a "boundary bubble" where children decide what they allow and don't allow within their bubble.

Role-play Activity: Act out different scenarios (appropriate for the age group) where children can practice saying "No."

Label how each one of the five senses, saying how each helps you know when something is wrong or makes you uncomfortable

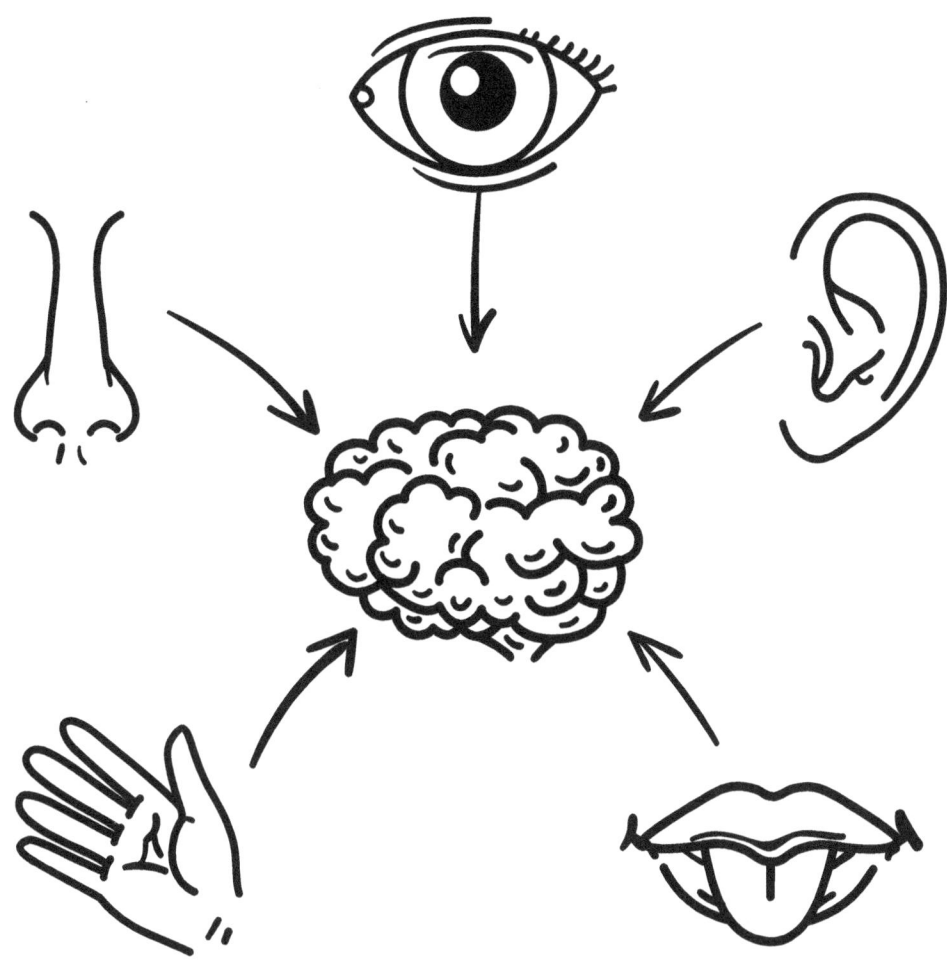

Week 3:
Saying "No" with Confidence

Objective:
- Empower students to confidently say "No" and trust their instincts.
- Children discover that they are in control of their bodies and empower them to say "No" confidently in uncomfortable situations.

Activity:
- Read and focus on the repeated phrase: "No Way, No How, I Say No!"

Discussion Questions:
- How do you feel when you say "No" to someone?
- What should you do if someone doesn't listen to your "No"?
- Why is it important to say "No" when something makes you feel uncomfortable?
- How can we practice saying "No"?

Activity:
- Create a confidence chant based on the book's verse that the class can recite together.
- Role-play scenarios where children practice saying "No" in different situations (e.g., someone trying to hug them when they don't want a hug)

Group Activity: Partner students to practice saying "No" in different scenarios where their boundaries might be challenged. Reinforce that it's okay to say no without feeling guilty.

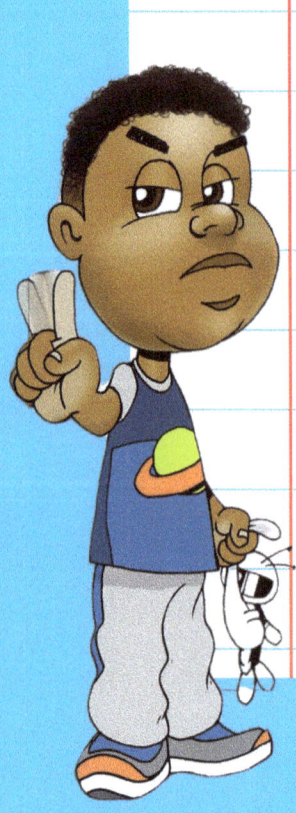

Week 4:
Private Parts & Respect

Objective:
- Understand what private parts are and why it's important to keep them private.
- Explain the difference between safe and unsafe touches and encourage children to trust their feelings when something feels wrong.

Activity: Use the book's verses about private parts as a guide for discussion.

Discussion Questions:
- What are private parts, and why is it important to keep them private?
- What is meant by respect?
- How do you feel when someone respects your boundaries?
- How do you feel when someone respects your boundaries about your private parts?
- What is a safe touch? What is an unsafe touch?
- What can you do if someone touches you in a way that doesn't feel right?

Activity:
- "Draw the Line" exercise: Children use red markers to draw lines on a diagram showing where private parts are and how they want to protect their boundaries.
- "Safe or Unsafe?" game: Present different scenarios and ask children if they are safe or unsafe.
- Create a "Feelings Chart" where children can draw or write how certain touches make them feel.

Homework: Write or draw an example of how you would tell a trusted adult if someone makes you feel uncomfortable.

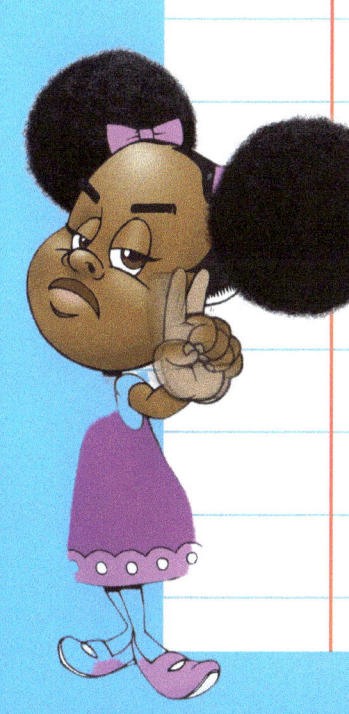

Is this safe or unsafe?
A teacher asks for a high-five in front of the class.

Is this safe or unsafe?
A neighbor invites you to come inside their house without telling your parents.

Is this safe or unsafe?
A stranger at the park offers you candy and says, "Don't tell your parents."

Is this safe or unsafe?
A friend asks you to look at a picture on their phone, but you feel unsure about it.

Is this safe or unsafe?
A teacher asks for a high-five in front of the class.

Is this safe or unsafe?
An older sibling gives you a hug when you feel sad, and you're okay with it.

QUESTIONS TO ASK:
- What would you do if someone asks you to keep a secret that makes you feel uncomfortable?
- How can you tell if a situation feels unsafe?
- What should you do if a stranger offers you a ride or gift?
- Who are trusted adults you can go to if you feel unsafe?
- What are some ways to say "no" if someone makes you uncomfortable?

STATEMENTS TO DISCUSS

- "It's okay to say no to hugs or touches, even from people you know."
    - Ask: Why is it important to say no if you don't feel comfortable?
- "Always check with your parents before going somewhere with someone."
    - Ask: Why do you think it's important to let your parents or guardians know where you are?
- "Secrets about surprises, like a birthday party, are okay. Secrets that make you feel worried are not."
    - Ask: Can you give an example of a good secret and a bad secret?
- "You don't have to do anything that feels wrong, even if someone says they are your friend."
    - Ask: How would you respond if a friend asks you to do something unsafe?
- "Your body belongs to you, and you decide who touches it."
    - Ask: What would you do if someone touches you in a way you don't like?

SCENARIO ANSWERS:

Scenario: A teacher asks for a high-five in front of the class.
Answer: Safe. High-fives are appropriate, especially in public spaces.

Scenario: A neighbor invites you to come inside their house without telling your parents.
Answer: Unsafe. Always let your parents or guardians know where you are going.

Scenario: A stranger at the park offers you candy and says, "Don't tell your parents."
Answer: Unsafe. You should not take things from strangers, especially if they tell you to keep it a secret.

Scenario: A friend asks you to look at a picture on their phone, but you feel unsure about it.
Answer: Unsafe. If something feels wrong, it's okay to say no and tell an adult.

Scenario: An older sibling gives you a hug when you feel sad, and you're okay with it.
Answer: Safe. This is appropriate if you feel comfortable.

Week 5:
Building a Safety Plan

Objective: Equip children with a plan of action if they ever feel unsafe or uncomfortable.

Activity: Discuss how the characters in the book use their voices and senses to protect themselves.

Discussion Questions:
- Who are safe adults you can go to if something happens?
- What are the steps you can take if you feel uncomfortable or unsafe?

Activity: Have students create their own "Safety Plan" booklet, outlining what they would do in an uncomfortable situation and who they would talk to.

Group Discussion:
- Reinforce that it's always okay to speak up and that they should never be afraid to tell a trusted adult.
- What should you do if you feel uncomfortable in a situation?
- Who can you talk to if something feels wrong?

Encourage children to listen to their inner voice and understand that their feelings matter.

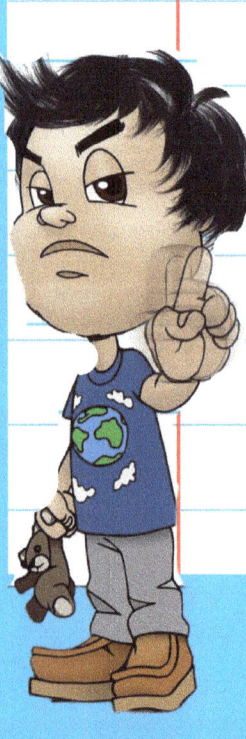

Activity:
- Draw a picture of a trusted adult in your life that you can talk to if you ever feel unsafe.
- Practice saying "No" and "Stop" firmly, and role-play scenarios where they go to a trusted adult for help.

My Safety Plan

Create your own "Safety Plan" booklet, outlining what you would do in an uncomfortable situation and who you would talk to.

My Trusted Adult

- Draw a picture of a trusted adult in your life that you can talk to if you ever feel unsafe.
- Practice saying "No" and "Stop" firmly, and role-play scenarios where you go to a trusted adult for help.

Week 6:
Conclusion & Celebration of Boundaries

Objective: Celebrate the children's understanding of their right to say "No" and reinforce lessons learned.

Activity: Hold a "Celebration of Boundaries" party where each child shares something they learned about body safety.

Reflection Activity: Have students write or draw a personal pledge about respecting their own body and others.

Final Activity: Create a class book titled "We Say No" where each student contributes a page about how they will use the lessons from the book in their daily lives.

Ongoing Activities:
- Weekly Reflection: Continue discussing boundaries and body safety throughout the year by having weekly reflection moments where children can share their experiences or thoughts.
- Parent Involvement: Send home weekly discussion prompts for parents to reinforce body safety conversations at home.

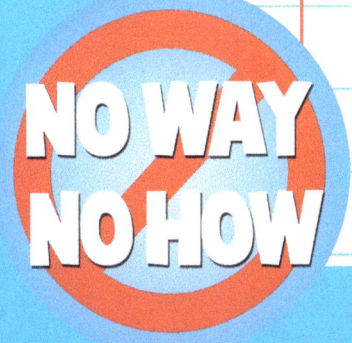

My Pledge Card

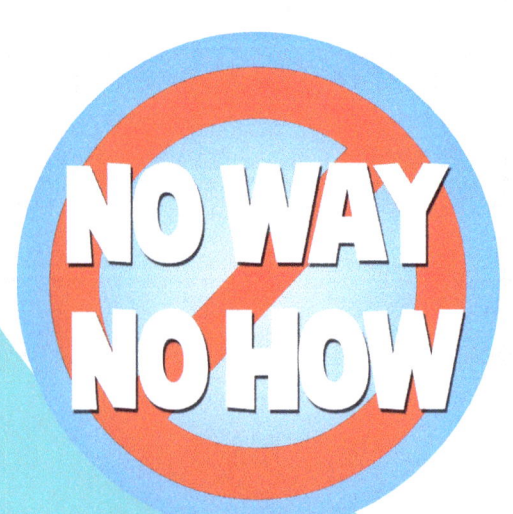
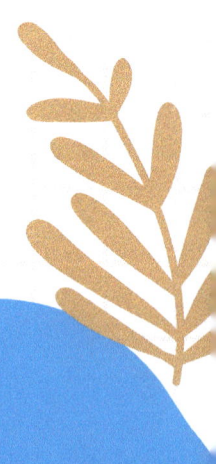

Give children the following Body Safety Quiz to assess their understanding of safe versus unsafe behaviors and the importance of saying "No" when they feel uncomfortable.

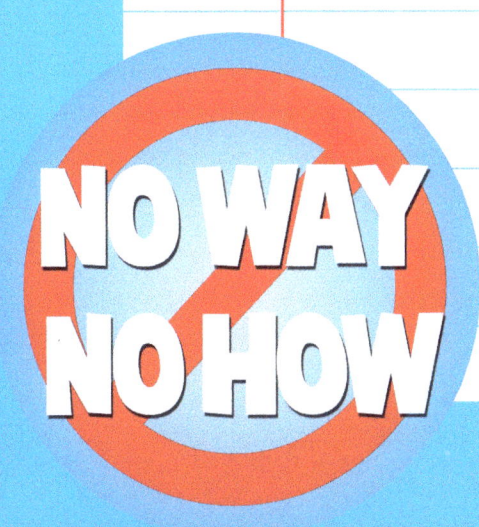

Body Safety Quiz

Complete this assessment of your understanding of safe vs. unsafe behaviors and the importance of saying "No" when you feel uncomfortable.

Circle the best answer for each question.

1. What should you do if someone touches you in a way that makes you feel uncomfortable?
    A. Keep it a secret.
    B. Tell a trusted adult.
    C. Ignore it.

2. Is it okay for someone to touch your private parts if they say it's a game?
    A. Yes, if they are a friend.
    B. No, because it's your body, and you say who can touch it.
    C. Only if you feel like playing.

3. Who are the safe adults you can go to if something doesn't feel right? (Circle all that apply)
    A. Parents
    B. Teachers
    C. Strangers
    D. Siblings

4. If someone asks you to keep a secret about touching, what should you do?
    A. Keep the secret because they asked you to.
    B. Say "No" and tell an adult you trust.
    C. Wait until you feel like telling someone later.

5. Which of these is an example of a safe touch?
    A. A high-five from a friend.
    B. Someone trying to touch your private parts.
    C. A hug when you don't want one.

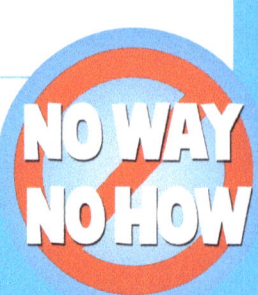

6. If you don't want to hug someone, what should you do?
    A. Say "No, thank you," or "I don't want to."
    B. Hug them anyway so they don't get mad.
    C. Run away and hide.

7. What should you say if someone shows you pictures of private parts?
    A. Say "No" and tell an adult.
    B. Look at them but don't tell anyone.
    C. Tell your friends about it.

8. True or False: It's okay to say "No" if someone asks you to do something that makes you uncomfortable.
    A. True
    B. False

9. What should you do if someone touches you and then says you'll get in trouble if you tell?
    A. Don't tell anyone so you don't get in trouble.
    B. Tell an adult you trust right away.
    C. Try to forget about it.

10. How do you feel when you say "No" to something that doesn't feel right?

Write about a time when you said "No" to someone. How did it make you feel? How can saying "No" help keep you safe?

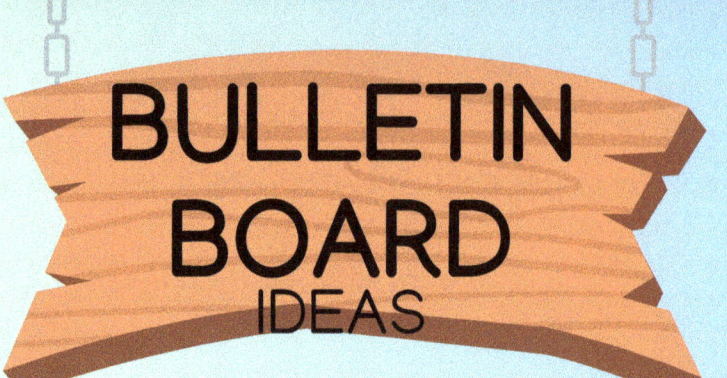

BULLETIN BOARD IDEAS

SCHOOLS & COMMUNITY CENTERS

My Body, My Rules

- Display cutouts of hands with empowering phrases like "I Have the Right to Say No!"
- Include a section with trusted adults' names and resources for children who need help.

Safe or Unsafe? Let's Learn Together

- Interactive board with different scenarios where students can attach answers under "Safe" or "Unsafe."
- Provide response tips for each scenario.

Trusted Adults: Who Can I Talk To?

- Showcase pictures or drawings of trusted adults (teachers, counselors, parents, clergy) children can turn to for help.
- Add a "What Makes Someone a Trusted Adult?" section.

Ways to Say No!

- Display speech bubbles with different ways to assert boundaries:
  - "No, I don't like that."
  - "Stop, that makes me uncomfortable."
  - "I need to tell an adult."

Your Five Senses Keep You Safe

- Create a sensory-themed board showing how sight, hearing, touch, taste, and smell help us recognize danger.
- Include real-life examples, like "If you see something that makes you uncomfortable, tell an adult."

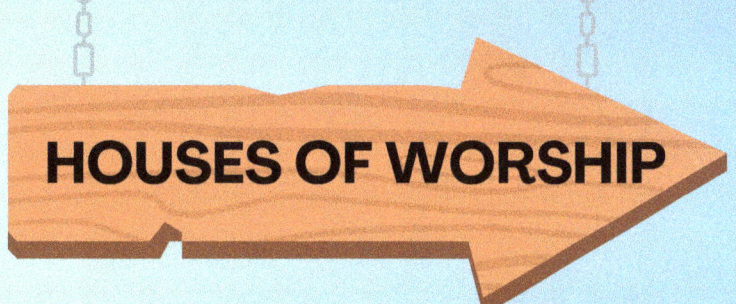

HOUSES OF WORSHIP

BULLETIN BOARD IDEAS

Safe & Supportive Spaces
- Share helpline numbers and trusted community members children can turn to.
- Include a prayer or affirmation about safety and well-being.

Respecting Boundaries is a Value We Share
- Highlight teachings from religious texts about respect, kindness, and protection.
- Include affirmations such as "My body is a trust, and I will keep it safe."

What to Do If You Feel Unsafe
- Display steps to follow if a child feels unsafe:
    - Say "No"
    - Move away
    - Tell a trusted adult
    - Keep telling until you are heard

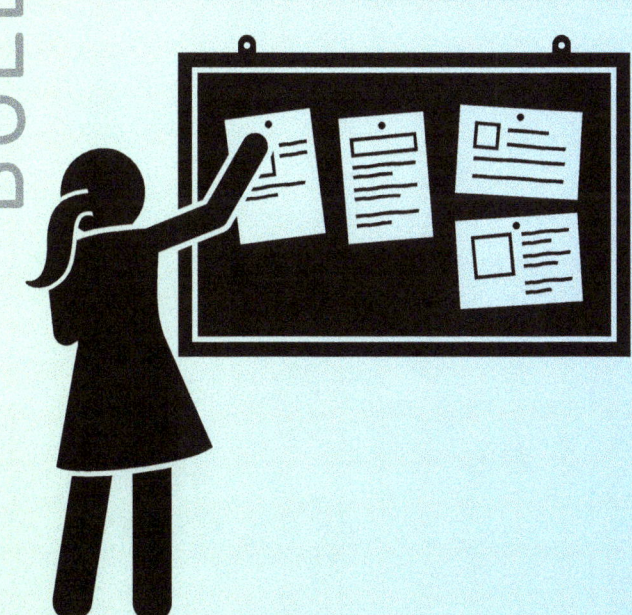

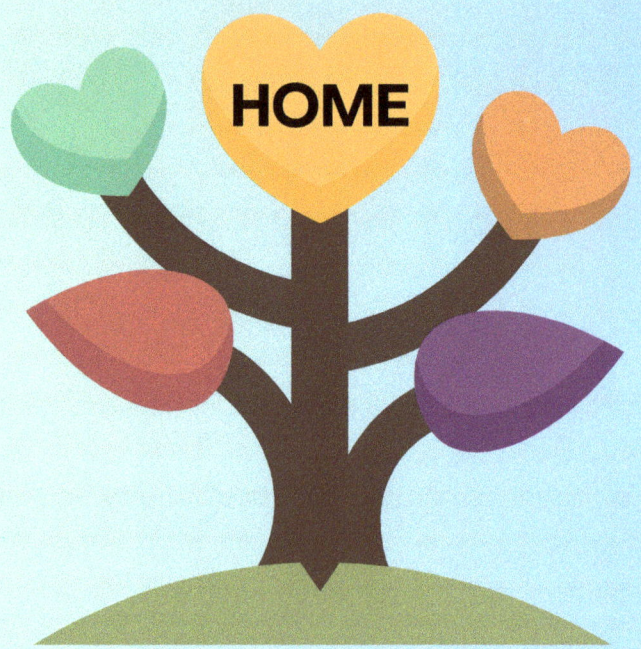

BULLETIN BOARD IDEAS

No Way, No How, I Say No!" Wall

- Let children write or draw ways they feel empowered to say "No" in different situations.

Who Are My Trusted Adults

- Family members write down their names so children always know who to go to if they need help.
- These bulletin board ideas help reinforce body safety, personal boundaries, and self-advocacy in a visual, engaging way.

Family Safety Rules

- Post clear rules about body safety (e.g., "We do not keep unsafe secrets," "No one should touch our private areas").
- Have children help decorate with drawings and stickers.

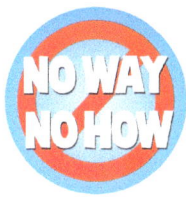

Guidelines for Developing a Child Safety and Abuse Prevention Policy

Policies are essential because they provide a clear, structured approach to ensuring the safety and well-being of children in any environment they frequent, such as schools, houses of worship, or community centers.

Developing and implementing these policies demonstrates a deep understanding of the immense responsibility you carry as a guardian or caretaker. These guidelines serve as a legal and ethical safeguard as well as a proactive measure to create a culture of trust, accountability, and vigilance.

By establishing clear protocols, you are protecting children from potential harm, and you are reinforcing the confidence that families, staff, and the community place in your ability to provide a safe, nurturing environment for every child in your care.

1. Define the Purpose and Scope
- Clearly state why the policy is necessary and who it applies to (e.g., staff, volunteers, educators, clergy, and community members).
- Emphasize a zero-tolerance stance on abuse and a commitment to child protection.

2. Conduct Research & Ensure Legal Compliance
- Review state, federal, and religious guidelines on child protection and mandatory reporting.
- Consult child protection agencies, legal advisors, and community stakeholders.
- Reference best practices from similar organizations.

3. Structure the Policy with Key Sections
- A well-organized policy should include:
    - Introduction & Purpose – Commitment to child safety.
    - Definitions – Types of abuse (physical, emotional, sexual, neglect).
    - Screening & Hiring Policies – Background checks and reference verification.
    - Training & Education – Annual staff training on abuse prevention and reporting.
    - Safe Environment & Conduct Guidelines – Rules for adult-child interactions and supervision.
    - Mandatory Reporting Procedures – Steps for reporting suspected abuse.
    - Response Plan – Actions to take when an allegation arises.
    - Facility Safety & Supervision – Security measures and check-in/check-out procedures.
    - Parent & Community Involvement – Education and resources for families.
    - Policy Review & Updates – Frequency of updates and responsible parties.

4. Ensure Practicality & Enforceability
- Use clear, simple language for accessibility.
- Provide real-life examples to clarify appropriate vs. inappropriate behavior.
- Include reporting contacts and emergency numbers.

5. Communicate & Train Staff, Volunteers, & Parents
- Require annual child safety training for all personnel.
- Make the policy easily accessible (printed copies, website, handbook).
- Conduct information sessions to educate parents and community members.

6. Review & Update Regularly
- Conduct annual policy reviews to incorporate new laws and best practices.
- Allow feedback from staff, parents, and children for continuous improvement.

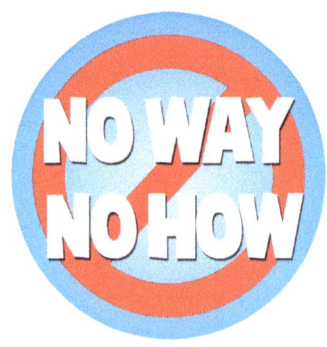

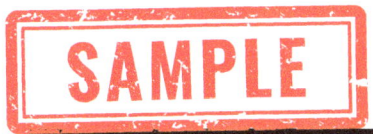

School Child Safety Policy

The school is dedicated to creating an environment where every child can learn, grow, and thrive without fear of harm. By following the guidelines set forth in this policy, we can work together to ensure that all students are protected and safe within our school community.

Scope: This policy applies to all employees, volunteers, contractors, and visitors of the school, as well as to any third-party organizations involved in activities within the school premises.

1. Commitment to Child Safety - The school is committed to providing a safe and supportive environment for all students. We recognize our duty of care to protect children from harm, both within and outside the classroom, and to promote their physical, emotional, and mental well-being.

2. Child Protection Procedures
- Reporting Concerns: All staff members are required to report any suspicion of child abuse or neglect to the designated Child Protection Officer (CPO) immediately. Reports can be made confidentially, and all reports will be treated seriously and investigated thoroughly.
- Mandatory Reporting: In accordance with local laws, staff members are obligated to report any suspected or confirmed cases of abuse to the appropriate authorities.
- Background Checks: All staff members, volunteers, and contractors undergo comprehensive background checks to ensure that they are fit to work with children.
- Training: All employees and volunteers receive regular child protection training, including recognizing the signs of abuse and the procedures for reporting concerns.

3. Code of Conduct for Interactions with Children
To prevent any inappropriate interactions, the school has established the following guidelines:
- Physical Contact: Physical contact with students should only occur when necessary and appropriate, such as to assist with personal care or provide comfort in distressing situations. Any contact should be done respectfully and professionally.
- One-on-One Interactions: All one-on-one interactions between staff and students should be conducted in open and visible areas. Private meetings should be avoided unless absolutely necessary and should be documented.
- Communication: Any communication with students (including via social media) should be professional, appropriate, and consistent with the school's values. Personal relationships outside of school should not be fostered.

4. Safe Environment and Supervision - Safe Facilities: The school is responsible for maintaining safe facilities, including secure entry points, classrooms, and play areas. All safety hazards should be identified and addressed immediately.
Adequate Supervision: Children will be supervised at all times while in school or during school-sponsored activities. The ratio of staff to students will meet or exceed recommended standards.

5. Addressing Allegations of Abuse or Neglect - Investigation: Any allegation of abuse or neglect will be taken seriously and promptly investigated by the designated CPO, in collaboration with appropriate authorities.
- Support for Victims: The school will provide counseling and support services to students who are victims of abuse or neglect, ensuring their emotional and psychological well-being.
- Confidentiality: All parties involved in an investigation will be treated with dignity and respect. The confidentiality of the child and the parties involved will be maintained, as much as possible, within legal and procedural boundaries.

6. Roles and Responsibilities - Designated Child Protection Officer (CPO): The CPO is responsible for overseeing child protection procedures, ensuring that staff members are properly trained, and acting as the point of contact for any safety concerns or incidents.
- Staff and Volunteers: All staff and volunteers are responsible for adhering to this policy, maintaining vigilance for signs of abuse or neglect, and promptly reporting any concerns.
- Parents and Guardians: The school encourages open communication with parents and guardians to ensure the safety of their children. Parents are encouraged to report any concerns to school officials.

7. Review and Evaluation - The Child Safety Policy will be reviewed annually to ensure that it remains effective and up-to-date with current laws and best practices. Any revisions will be communicated to all staff members, volunteers, and parents.

Signature of School Administrator: _____   Date: _____

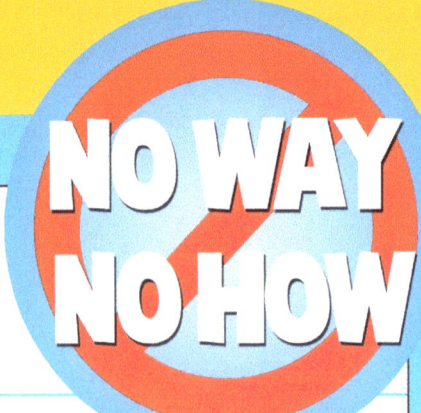
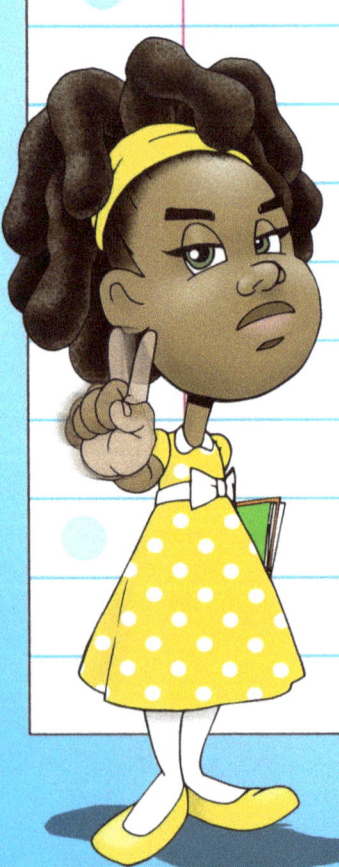

If you are a child or concerned about a child being abused call
1 (800) 422-4453

NO WAY NO HOW

Thank you!

Thank you for reading the book "No Way, No How, I Say No! by Dr. Qiana A. Johnson. And, thank you for taking time to really study the themes and main points of the book. Thank you for helping children to feel safe, to be empowered, and to recognize how to use their senses to keep themselves safe.

Answer Key:
1. B
2. B
3. A, B, D
4. B
5. A
6. A
7. A
8. A
9. B

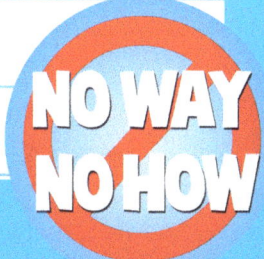

Resources

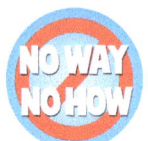

Teaching children about body safety and preventing child sexual abuse is crucial for their well-being. Here are some recommended resources, including websites, videos, and literature, to assist in this important education:

Websites:
- Educate2Empower Publishing: Offers a comprehensive guide titled "Body Safety Education" for parents, caregivers, and educators to protect children from sexual abuse. (E2E Publishing - https://e2epublishing.info)
- National Sexual Violence Resource Center (NSVRC): Provides resources focused on preventing child sexual abuse, including educational materials and statistics. (NSVRC
- Child Safety Resources: Developed to support adults in having age-appropriate conversations with children about body safety and sexual abuse. (Child Safety
- Enough Abuse Campaign: Offers prevention education resources aimed at stopping child sexual abuse through community education and awareness. (Enough Abuse)
- Nurtured First – The Body Safety Toolkit: Provides scripts, games, and activities to help teach body safety and consent to children. (Nurtured First)
- Darkness to Light: Features a range of training programs for adults to prevent child sexual abuse and protect children. (D2L
- Kidpower: Offers resources for schools and parents to protect children and teens from sexual abuse, bullying, and abduction. (Kidpower

Videos:
- "My Superhero Voice" Storybook Video: A culturally inclusive storybook that helps adults start conversations with children about body safety. (Child Safety
- Lauren's Kids – Safer, Smarter Kids Program: Provides educational videos as part of a comprehensive curriculum teaching children safety tools. (Lauren's Kids

Literature:
- "Body Safety Education" by Jayneen Sanders: A step-by-step guide for parents and educators on protecting children from sexual abuse through body safety education. (E2E Publishing
- "My Body! What I Say Goes!" by Jayneen Sanders: A children's book that empowers kids to understand body autonomy and assert their rights.
- "I Said No! A Kid-to-Kid Guide to Keeping Private Parts Private" by Kimberly King: Uses a simple, straightforward approach to teach children about setting boundaries.
- "Some Secrets Should Never Be Kept" by Jayneen Sanders: A storybook that sensitively broaches the subject of keeping children safe from inappropriate touch.
- Harper Learns Body Boundaries: Teaching Kids Consent, Respecting Personal Space, Private Parts Safety, When To Speak Up And Say No, And Social Life Skills (Enabling Kids To Thrive) by Pang Guerrero and Liz Scofield | Jun 25, 2023
-

These resources provide valuable tools for educating children about body safety and preventing child sexual abuse. It's important to review each resource to ensure it aligns with your educational goals and is appropriate for the children's age and comprehension levels.

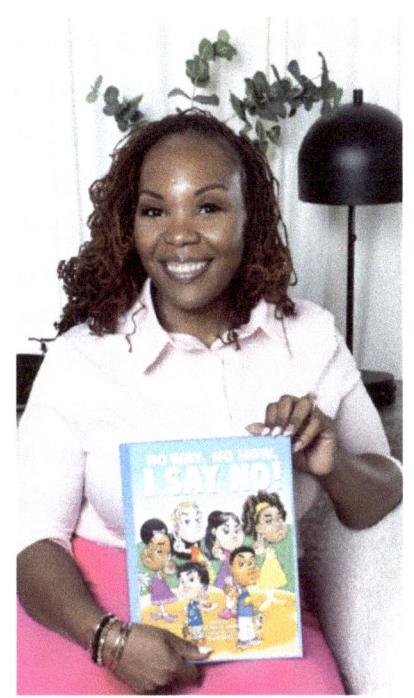

Dr. Qiana A. Johnson is an accomplished Family Nurse Practitioner, forensic nurse, educator, and advocate for child and adolescent health and safety. She earned her Doctor of Nursing Practice from the University of Tennessee Health Science Center in 2014, specializing in Family and Forensic Nursing. With over 15 years of professional experience, Dr. Johnson's expertise spans pediatric care, forensic nursing, and sexual assault examination. She owns and is a provider at Lotus Wellness and Aesthetics. She has also worked with Children's Healthcare of Atlanta in the Child Advocacy Center. Her teaching roles include serving as an adjunct professor at Chamberlain College of Nursing. Dr. Johnson is a sought-after speaker on topics such as child abuse, sexual assault, and STI prevention. Her scholarly work includes presenting at national conferences and publishing studies on adolescent sexual assault. Through her work, Dr. Johnson combines clinical expertise and compassionate care to empower individuals, educate communities, and advocate for justice and safety for children and families.

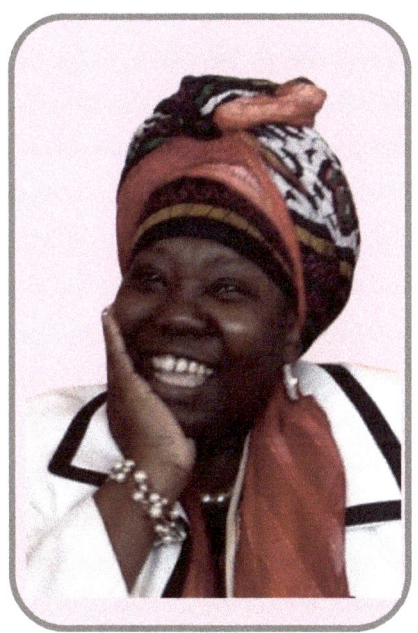

Qur'an Shakir is a seasoned Master Educator with over 40 years of experience shaping young minds and empowering communities. As an author, curriculum developer, and workshop presenter, she is dedicated to creating meaningful learning experiences that inspire growth and self-discovery. A passionate advocate for youth, she trains children to use their voices with confidence and equips educators with tools to foster engaged, empowered learners. Known as a teacher of teachers, Qur'an Shakir's work extends beyond the classroom, impacting communities through leadership, advocacy, and transformative education. Her commitment to holistic well-being and personal development is reflected in her writing, workshops, and innovative programs designed to uplift individuals of all ages.

www.ingramcontent.com/pod-product-compliance
Lightning Source LLC
Chambersburg PA
CBHW042359030426
42337CB00032B/5153